CONTENTS

CHAPTER 1: INTRODUCTION TO PELVIC FLOOR MUSCLES

The pelvic floor muscles, often overlooked and underestimated, are a crucial group of muscles that play a vital role in the health and function of the lower abdomen. Located at the base of the pelvis, these muscles stretch like a hammock from the pubic bone at the front to the tailbone at the back. They support the bladder, bowel, and, in men, the prostate, helping to maintain control over urinary and bowel functions and contributing to sexual health.

Importance of Pelvic Floor Muscles

1. Bladder Control: One of the primary functions of the pelvic floor muscles is to support the bladder. These muscles help control the release of urine by contracting and relaxing. Weak pelvic floor muscles can lead to urinary incontinence, where there is involuntary leakage of urine. Strengthening these muscles can significantly improve bladder control.

2. Bowel Control: Just like with the bladder, the pelvic floor muscles also play a critical role in bowel control. They support the rectum and help manage the passage of stool. Strengthening the pelvic floor can prevent issues such as fecal incontinence and support overall digestive

health.

3. Sexual Health: The pelvic floor muscles contribute to sexual function and satisfaction. Strong pelvic floor muscles can enhance erections and contribute to better control during ejaculation. They also play a role in the sensation during sexual activity, making them essential for sexual health and enjoyment.

4. Support of Abdominal Organs: The pelvic floor muscles provide a foundation for the abdominal organs, supporting their proper position and function. This support is crucial for maintaining overall abdominal health and preventing organ prolapse.

Why Keep Pelvic Floor Muscles Strong?

Maintaining strong pelvic floor muscles is not just about preventing problems; it's about enhancing overall quality of life. Here are some reasons why you should focus on strengthening these muscles:

- Prevention of Incontinence: By keeping your pelvic floor muscles strong, you can prevent urinary and fecal incontinence, which can be embarrassing and significantly impact your daily life.

- Improved Sexual Function: Strong pelvic floor muscles can enhance sexual performance and satisfaction, contributing to a healthier and more fulfilling sex life.

- Support During Physical Activities: These muscles provide essential support during physical activities, including lifting, running, and other exercises, reducing the risk of injury and improving performance.

- Recovery from Surgery or Injury: For those who have undergone surgery or experienced injuries affecting the pelvic region, strengthening the pelvic floor muscles can aid in recovery and improve overall outcomes.

How to Identify Your Pelvic Floor Muscles

Before you start any pelvic floor exercises, it's essential to identify the correct muscles. Here are a few simple ways to locate them:

- Stopping the Flow of Urine: While urinating, try to stop the flow of urine midstream. The muscles you use to do this are your pelvic floor muscles. However, do this only to identify the muscles, not as a regular exercise, as it can lead to urinary problems.

- Tightening the Muscles to Prevent Passing Gas: Imagine you are trying to prevent yourself from passing gas. The muscles you tighten are your pelvic floor muscles.

Understanding the location and function of these muscles is the first step towards strengthening them and reaping the benefits of a healthy pelvic floor. In the following chapters, we will explore various exercises and techniques to help you maintain strong and healthy pelvic floor muscles.

CHAPTER 2: BENEFITS OF PELVIC FLOOR EXERCISES

Pelvic floor exercises, often referred to as Kegel exercises, offer a wide range of benefits that contribute significantly to overall well-being. By strengthening the pelvic floor muscles, you can improve various bodily functions and enhance your quality of life. This chapter details the primary benefits of pelvic floor exercises and how they positively impact health.

Improved Bladder Control

One of the most significant benefits of pelvic floor exercises is improved bladder control. Strong pelvic floor muscles help:

- **Prevent Urinary Incontinence**: Involuntary leakage of urine can occur due to weak pelvic floor muscles. Regular exercises strengthen these muscles, reducing the risk of urinary incontinence.

- **Reduce Urgency and Frequency**: Strengthening the pelvic floor can help control the urge to urinate and reduce the frequency of trips to the bathroom, especially at night.

- **Support During High-Impact Activities**: For those who engage in high-impact sports or activities, a strong pelvic floor helps prevent stress incontinence, where urine leaks due to pressure on the bladder from activities like running or jumping.

Enhanced Bowel Control

Pelvic floor exercises also play a crucial role in maintaining bowel control. Benefits include:

- **Prevention of Fecal Incontinence**: Strengthened pelvic floor muscles help prevent the involuntary leakage of stool, providing better control over bowel movements.

- **Improved Digestive Health**: A strong pelvic floor supports the proper functioning of the bowels, aiding in smoother and more regular bowel movements.

Enhanced Sexual Function

For men, pelvic floor exercises can significantly enhance sexual function. Benefits include:

- **Improved Erectile Function**: Strong pelvic floor muscles contribute to better blood flow to the penis, which can improve erections and help with erectile dysfunction.

- **Better Control During Ejaculation**: Strengthening these muscles can provide better control over ejaculation, potentially extending the duration of sexual activity.

- **Increased Sexual Satisfaction**: Many men report heightened sensation and satisfaction during sex after regularly performing pelvic floor exercises.

Reduced Risk of Prolapse

Pelvic organ prolapse occurs when pelvic organs, such as the bladder or rectum, descend into the vaginal area due to weakened pelvic floor muscles. Pelvic floor exercises help by:

- **Providing Support to Pelvic Organs**: Strong muscles offer better support to the pelvic organs, reducing the risk of prolapse.

- **Aiding in Prolapse Management**: For those already experiencing mild prolapse, pelvic floor exercises can help manage and alleviate symptoms.

Improved Core Stability and Posture

The pelvic floor is a crucial part of the core muscle group, which includes the abdominal muscles, lower back muscles, and diaphragm. Benefits include:

- **Enhanced Core Stability**: A strong pelvic floor contributes to overall core strength, improving balance and stability.

- **Better Posture**: Strengthening the pelvic floor muscles supports a healthy posture by maintaining proper alignment of the pelvis and spine.

Support During Pregnancy and Postpartum Recovery

For men, while pregnancy is not relevant, these exercises can still offer benefits if they are part of a family supporting a partner through pregnancy and postpartum recovery:

- **Supporting Partner's Health**: Understanding and practicing pelvic floor exercises can help men support their partners better during pregnancy and postpartum recovery.

- **Increased Awareness of Pelvic Health**: Men can benefit from increased awareness and knowledge of pelvic health, which is crucial for overall well-being.

Overall Well-being and Confidence

Engaging in regular pelvic floor exercises can also lead to improved overall well-being:

- **Increased Confidence**: Better control over bladder and bowel functions can significantly boost confidence in social and professional settings.

- **Enhanced Quality of Life**: Improved physical health, sexual satisfaction, and reduced risk of incontinence all contribute to a better quality of life.

How to Measure Progress

Tracking your progress can be motivating and help ensure you are performing the exercises correctly. Consider:

- **Keeping a Journal**: Record the frequency and duration of your exercises, along with any noticeable improvements in bladder or bowel control.

- **Seeking Professional Guidance**: A physical therapist or healthcare provider can help assess your progress and provide additional guidance if needed.

In conclusion, the benefits of pelvic floor exercises extend beyond just physical health. They contribute to improved mental well-being, confidence, and overall quality of life. By incorporating these exercises into your daily routine, you can experience significant improvements in various aspects of your health and well-being.

CHAPTER 3: UNDERSTANDING THE PELVIC FLOOR

Before starting pelvic floor exercises, it's essential to understand the anatomy and function of the pelvic floor. Having a clear picture of what these muscles are and how they work will help you perform the exercises correctly and effectively. This chapter provides a simple explanation of the structure and role of the pelvic floor muscles.

Anatomy of the Pelvic Floor

The pelvic floor is a group of muscles and connective tissues located at the base of your pelvis. It stretches like a hammock from the pubic bone (at the front) to the tailbone (at the back) and from one sitting bone to the other. Here's a breakdown of its key components:

- **Levator Ani Muscles**: This group of muscles includes the pubococcygeus, puborectalis, and iliococcygeus. These muscles are primarily responsible for supporting the pelvic organs and controlling the opening and closing of the urethra and anus.

- **Coccygeus Muscle**: This muscle works alongside the levator ani muscles to support the pelvic organs and stabilize the coccyx (tailbone).

- **Perineal Muscles**: These are the muscles found between

the scrotum and anus. They play a role in supporting the pelvic organs and are involved in sexual function.

Functions of the Pelvic Floor

The pelvic floor muscles have several crucial functions:

1. **Support of Pelvic Organs**
   - The pelvic floor muscles support the bladder, rectum, and, in men, the prostate. They help keep these organs in place and ensure they function correctly.

2. **Control of Bladder and Bowel**
   - The muscles control the release of urine and feces by contracting and relaxing around the urethra and anus. They allow you to start and stop the flow of urine and control bowel movements.

3. **Sexual Function**
   - The pelvic floor muscles play an essential role in sexual function. They help achieve and maintain erections and control ejaculation. Strong pelvic floor muscles can enhance sexual sensation and satisfaction.

4. **Stability and Support of the Core**
   - The pelvic floor muscles are a vital part of the core muscle group, which includes the abdominal muscles, diaphragm, and lower back muscles. They work together to provide stability and support to the spine and pelvis.

How the Pelvic Floor Works

The pelvic floor muscles are like any other muscle group in your body: they can be strengthened through regular exercise and can become weak if not used. Here's how they work:

- **Contraction**: When you contract your pelvic floor

muscles, they lift and tighten. This action supports the pelvic organs, closes the openings of the urethra and anus, and helps control the release of urine and feces.

- **Relaxation**: When you relax your pelvic floor muscles, they lengthen and release. This action allows the bladder and bowel to empty and supports the normal functioning of the pelvic organs.

Identifying Your Pelvic Floor Muscles

Before you can start exercising your pelvic floor muscles, you need to be able to identify them. Here are a couple of simple ways to locate your pelvic floor muscles:

- **Stopping the Flow of Urine**: The next time you urinate, try to stop the flow of urine midstream. The muscles you use to do this are your pelvic floor muscles. Only use this method to identify the muscles, not as a regular exercise, as it can lead to urinary problems.

- **Tightening to Prevent Passing Gas**: Imagine you are trying to stop yourself from passing gas. The muscles you tighten are your pelvic floor muscles.

Common Issues with the Pelvic Floor

Several factors can weaken the pelvic floor muscles, leading to various issues. Some common causes of pelvic floor weakness include:

- **Aging**: As you age, your muscles naturally weaken, including the pelvic floor muscles.

- **Surgery or Injury**: Surgeries involving the prostate, bladder, or bowel, as well as injuries to the pelvic region, can weaken the pelvic floor muscles.

- **Chronic Coughing**: Conditions that cause chronic coughing, such as asthma or bronchitis, can strain the pelvic floor muscles over time.

- **Obesity**: Excess body weight puts additional pressure on the pelvic floor muscles, weakening them over time.

Understanding these factors can help you take proactive steps to strengthen and maintain your pelvic floor muscles.

The Importance of Regular Exercise

Just like any other muscle group, the pelvic floor muscles need regular exercise to stay strong and functional. Regular pelvic floor exercises can:

- **Prevent Incontinence**: Strengthening these muscles can prevent both urinary and fecal incontinence.

- **Enhance Sexual Health**: Strong pelvic floor muscles can improve erectile function and control over ejaculation.

- **Support Overall Core Stability**: By integrating pelvic floor exercises into your routine, you contribute to overall core strength and stability.

In the following chapters, we will explore specific exercises to strengthen your pelvic floor muscles and techniques to incorporate them into your daily routine. By understanding the anatomy and function of the pelvic floor, you are better equipped to perform these exercises effectively and achieve the best results.

CHAPTER 4: BASIC PELVIC FLOOR EXERCISES

In this chapter, we will introduce you to three fundamental pelvic floor exercises: Kegel Exercises, Quick Flick Kegels, and Long Hold Kegels. These exercises form the foundation of a pelvic floor workout routine, helping you build strength, endurance, and control over your pelvic floor muscles. By performing these exercises regularly and correctly, you can reap the numerous benefits discussed in previous chapters.

Kegel Exercises

Kegel exercises are the cornerstone of pelvic floor strengthening routines. They involve the repeated contraction and relaxation of the pelvic floor muscles. Here's how to perform them correctly:

Step-by-Step Guide:

1. **Identify the Pelvic Floor Muscles**: Before starting, ensure you know which muscles to target. Refer to Chapter 3 for identification techniques.

2. **Get Comfortable**: You can perform Kegels while sitting, standing, or lying down. Choose a position where you feel relaxed and comfortable.

3. **Contract the Muscles**: Slowly tighten your pelvic floor muscles as if you are trying to stop the flow of urine. Hold the contraction for 3-5 seconds.

4. **Relax the Muscles**: Gradually relax your muscles and rest for 3-5 seconds.

5. **Repeat**: Aim for 10-15 repetitions per session. Perform this exercise three times a day.

Tips for Effective Kegels:

- **Breathe Normally**: Do not hold your breath while performing the exercises.

- **Isolate the Muscles**: Avoid contracting your abdomen, buttocks, or thighs. Focus solely on your pelvic floor muscles.

- **Consistency is Key**: Regular practice is crucial for seeing results. Incorporate Kegels into your daily routine.

Quick Flick Kegels

Quick Flick Kegels involve rapid, short contractions of the pelvic floor muscles. This exercise helps build strength and endurance, improving your muscle response time.

Step-by-Step Guide:

1. **Identify the Pelvic Floor Muscles**: Ensure you know which muscles to target.

2. **Get Comfortable**: You can perform this exercise in any comfortable position.

3. **Quick Contraction**: Quickly tighten your pelvic floor muscles for 1 second.

4. **Quick Relaxation**: Immediately relax your muscles for 1 second.

5. **Repeat**: Aim for 20-30 repetitions per session. Perform this exercise two to three times a day.

Tips for Effective Quick Flick Kegels:

- **Stay Focused**: Concentrate on the quick contractions and relaxations.

- **Consistency**: Regular practice will enhance your muscle response time and endurance.

Long Hold Kegels

Long Hold Kegels involve holding the contraction of the pelvic floor muscles for an extended period. This exercise enhances muscle control and strength.

Step-by-Step Guide:

1. **Identify the Pelvic Floor Muscles**: Ensure you know which muscles to target.
2. **Get Comfortable**: Choose a position where you feel relaxed and comfortable.
3. **Contract the Muscles**: Slowly tighten your pelvic floor muscles and hold the contraction for 10 seconds.
4. **Relax the Muscles**: Gradually relax your muscles and rest for 10 seconds.
5. **Repeat**: Aim for 5-10 repetitions per session. Perform this exercise two to three times a day.

Tips for Effective Long Hold Kegels:

- **Breathe Normally**: Do not hold your breath during the exercise.
- **Stay Relaxed**: Ensure the rest of your body remains relaxed while performing the exercise.
- **Build Gradually**: If 10 seconds is too long initially, start with a shorter hold and gradually increase the duration as your muscles strengthen.

Combining the Exercises

To achieve the best results, incorporate all three types of Kegel exercises into your routine. A balanced approach will help you build strength, endurance, and control over your pelvic floor muscles. Here's a sample weekly routine:

Sample Weekly Routine:

- **Monday, Wednesday, Friday**:
    - Kegel Exercises: 10-15 repetitions, three times a day
    - Long Hold Kegels: 5-10 repetitions, two times a day

- **Tuesday, Thursday, Saturday**:
    - Quick Flick Kegels: 20-30 repetitions, two times a day
    - Long Hold Kegels: 5-10 repetitions, two times a day

- **Sunday**:
    - Rest day or light routine of your choice

Remember, consistency is crucial. By regularly performing these basic pelvic floor exercises, you will strengthen your pelvic floor muscles, leading to improved bladder and bowel control, enhanced sexual function, and overall better pelvic health.

CHAPTER 5: ADVANCED PELVIC FLOOR EXERCISES

Once you have mastered the basic pelvic floor exercises, it's time to incorporate more advanced movements that not only target the pelvic floor muscles but also engage other muscle groups. This chapter introduces three advanced pelvic floor exercises: Bridge Pose, Squats, and Split Tabletop. These exercises will help you build a stronger and more resilient pelvic floor while improving overall strength and stability.

Bridge Pose

The Bridge Pose is a powerful exercise that targets the pelvic floor along with the glutes and lower back muscles. It helps to strengthen the core and improve pelvic stability.

Step-by-Step Guide:

1. **Starting Position**: Lie on your back with your knees bent and feet flat on the floor, hip-width apart. Place your arms at your sides with palms facing down.

2. **Engage the Core and Pelvic Floor**: Tighten your pelvic floor muscles and engage your core by pulling your belly button towards your spine.

3. **Lift the Hips**: Press your feet into the floor and lift your hips towards the ceiling, creating a straight line from your shoulders to your knees. Hold the position for a few

seconds.

4. **Lower the Hips**: Slowly lower your hips back to the starting position, keeping your pelvic floor muscles engaged.

5. **Repeat**: Aim for 10-15 repetitions per session. Perform this exercise two to three times a day.

Tips for Effective Bridge Pose:

- **Breathe Deeply**: Inhale as you lift your hips and exhale as you lower them.

- **Avoid Overarching**: Ensure your back remains in a neutral position and avoid overarching your lower back.

- **Engage the Glutes**: Focus on squeezing your glutes as you lift your hips for maximum benefit.

Squats

Squats are a compound exercise that engages the pelvic floor muscles, thighs, and glutes. They provide a comprehensive workout that enhances strength and stability.

Step-by-Step Guide:

1. **Starting Position**: Stand with your feet shoulder-width apart and toes pointing slightly outward. Place your hands on your hips or extend them in front of you for balance.

2. **Engage the Core and Pelvic Floor**: Tighten your pelvic floor muscles and engage your core by pulling your belly button towards your spine.

3. **Lower into a Squat**: Bend your knees and lower your hips as if you are sitting back into a chair. Keep your chest lifted and your weight in your heels. Lower until your thighs are parallel to the floor or as far as your mobility allows.

4. **Rise Back Up**: Press through your heels to return to

the starting position, keeping your pelvic floor muscles engaged.

5. **Repeat**: Aim for 10-15 repetitions per session. Perform this exercise two to three times a day.

Tips for Effective Squats:

- **Maintain Proper Alignment**: Keep your knees in line with your toes and avoid letting them collapse inward.

- **Focus on Depth**: Lower your hips as far as your flexibility allows while maintaining good form.

- **Engage Multiple Muscles**: Ensure you are engaging your glutes, thighs, and pelvic floor throughout the movement.

Split Tabletop

The Split Tabletop is an advanced exercise that requires balance and engages multiple muscle groups, including the pelvic floor, core, and legs.

Step-by-Step Guide:

1. **Starting Position**: Begin on all fours with your hands directly under your shoulders and knees under your hips. Keep your back straight and your core engaged.

2. **Engage the Core and Pelvic Floor**: Tighten your pelvic floor muscles and engage your core by pulling your belly button towards your spine.

3. **Extend Opposite Arm and Leg**: Simultaneously extend your right arm forward and your left leg back, creating a straight line from your hand to your foot. Hold this position for a few seconds.

4. **Return to Starting Position**: Slowly return your arm and leg to the starting position, keeping your core and pelvic floor muscles engaged.

5. **Switch Sides**: Repeat the movement with your left arm

and right leg.

6. **Repeat**: Aim for 10-15 repetitions on each side per session. Perform this exercise two to three times a day.

Tips for Effective Split Tabletop:

- **Maintain Balance**: Focus on maintaining balance and stability throughout the movement.

- **Control the Movement**: Perform the exercise slowly and with control to engage the muscles effectively.

- **Avoid Sagging**: Keep your back straight and avoid letting your lower back sag.

Combining Advanced Exercises

To maximize the benefits of advanced pelvic floor exercises, incorporate all three into your routine. This balanced approach will help you build a stronger, more resilient pelvic floor and enhance overall strength and stability.

Sample Weekly Routine:

- **Monday, Wednesday, Friday**:
    - Bridge Pose: 10-15 repetitions, two times a day
    - Split Tabletop: 10-15 repetitions on each side, two times a day

- **Tuesday, Thursday, Saturday**:
    - Squats: 10-15 repetitions, two times a day
    - Split Tabletop: 10-15 repetitions on each side, two times a day

- **Sunday**:
    - Rest day or light routine of your choice

Remember, consistency and proper form are crucial for achieving the best results. By regularly performing these advanced pelvic floor exercises, you will strengthen your pelvic floor muscles, improve overall core stability, and enhance your physical health and well-being.

CHAPTER 6: INTEGRATING PELVIC FLOOR EXERCISES INTO DAILY LIFE

Consistency is key to reaping the long-term benefits of pelvic floor exercises. This chapter will guide you on how to seamlessly incorporate these exercises into your daily routine, ensuring that they become a natural part of your everyday activities.

Making Pelvic Floor Exercises a Habit

To make pelvic floor exercises a regular part of your life, you need to develop a habit. Here are some strategies to help you integrate these exercises into your daily routine:

1. **Set Reminders**: Use your phone, smartwatch, or a physical reminder (like a sticky note) to remind you to do your exercises. Set alarms or notifications at specific times each day.

2. **Associate with Daily Activities**: Link your exercises to activities you already do regularly. For example:
   - Perform Kegels while brushing your teeth in the morning and evening.
   - Do Bridge Poses before getting out of bed or going to sleep.
   - Practice Quick Flick Kegels while waiting at

traffic lights or during commercial breaks when watching TV.

3. **Start Small**: Begin with short, manageable sessions and gradually increase the duration and frequency as you become more comfortable with the exercises.

4. **Track Your Progress**: Keep a journal or use a mobile app to track your progress. Note the exercises you've done, the number of repetitions, and any improvements you've noticed. Tracking your progress can be motivating and help you stay committed.

Incorporating Exercises into Your Routine

Here's how you can fit pelvic floor exercises into different parts of your daily routine:

Morning Routine

- **Kegels with Breakfast Preparation**: While making breakfast or your morning coffee, perform a set of Kegels. This can be done discreetly and helps you start your day with a positive health habit.

- **Bridge Poses Before Work**: After waking up and before getting dressed, spend a few minutes doing Bridge Poses. This will activate your pelvic floor and core muscles, setting a good tone for the day.

During Work

- **Quick Flick Kegels at Your Desk**: While sitting at your desk, take a few moments every hour to perform Quick Flick Kegels. These can be done without anyone noticing and help keep your pelvic floor muscles engaged throughout the day.

- **Squats During Breaks**: Use your breaks to do a few squats. This not only strengthens your pelvic floor but also gets you moving and helps combat the effects of prolonged sitting.

Evening Routine

- **Long Hold Kegels While Watching TV**: During your evening relaxation time, such as while watching TV or reading, perform Long Hold Kegels. This helps integrate your exercises into a relaxing part of your day.

- **Bridge Poses Before Bed**: Incorporate a few Bridge Poses into your bedtime routine. This not only benefits your pelvic floor but also helps relax your lower back and prepare you for a restful sleep.

Exercise Integration with Other Physical Activities

You can also combine pelvic floor exercises with other physical activities you may already be doing:

- **Yoga**: Many yoga poses, like the Bridge Pose and other core-strengthening poses, naturally engage the pelvic floor muscles. Integrate these poses into your yoga routine to enhance pelvic floor strength.

- **Strength Training**: When performing exercises like deadlifts, lunges, or planks, focus on engaging your pelvic floor muscles. This will add an extra layer of benefit to your workouts.

- **Cardio Workouts**: Incorporate Quick Flick Kegels into your cardio routines, such as walking, running, or cycling. This can help maintain pelvic floor engagement even during aerobic activities.

Maintaining Motivation

Staying motivated is crucial for long-term success. Here are some tips to keep you motivated:

1. **Set Clear Goals**: Define what you want to achieve with your pelvic floor exercises. Whether it's improved bladder control, enhanced sexual function, or overall

core strength, having clear goals can keep you focused.

2. **Celebrate Progress**: Recognize and celebrate your achievements, no matter how small. Progress can be slow, but each step forward is a victory.

3. **Join a Community**: Consider joining a fitness or health community, either online or in person. Sharing your journey with others can provide support and encouragement.

Professional Guidance

If you're unsure about your technique or want to ensure you're performing the exercises correctly, seek professional guidance. A physical therapist or a fitness instructor with experience in pelvic health can provide personalized advice and help you refine your routine.

Sample Daily Routine

Here's a sample daily routine to help you visualize how to integrate pelvic floor exercises into your day:

- **Morning**:
  - Kegels while making breakfast (3-5 minutes)
  - Bridge Poses before getting dressed (5-10 minutes)

- **During Work**:
  - Quick Flick Kegels at your desk (1-2 minutes every hour)
  - Squats during morning and afternoon breaks (5 minutes each break)

- **Evening**:
  - Long Hold Kegels while watching TV (10 minutes)
  - Bridge Poses before bed (5-10 minutes)

By incorporating these exercises into your daily routine, you ensure consistency and long-term benefits. Regular practice will help you maintain strong, healthy pelvic floor muscles, enhancing your overall well-being and quality of life.

CHAPTER 7: COMMON MISTAKES AND HOW TO AVOID THEM

Performing pelvic floor exercises correctly is crucial for achieving the desired benefits. However, many people make common mistakes that can reduce the effectiveness of their workouts or even cause harm. This chapter identifies these common errors and provides tips on how to correct them for maximum effectiveness.

Mistake 1: Incorrect Muscle Engagement

Description: One of the most common mistakes is engaging the wrong muscles, such as the abdomen, buttocks, or thighs, instead of the pelvic floor muscles.

How to Avoid It:

- **Identify the Right Muscles**: Before starting, ensure you have correctly identified your pelvic floor muscles. Refer to Chapter 3 for identification techniques.

- **Isolate the Pelvic Floor**: Focus on contracting only the pelvic floor muscles. Place a hand on your abdomen and buttocks to ensure they remain relaxed.

- **Practice**: Practice isolating the pelvic floor muscles while lying down, as this position reduces the likelihood of engaging other muscles.

Mistake 2: Holding Your Breath

Description: Holding your breath while performing pelvic floor exercises can increase intra-abdominal pressure and reduce the effectiveness of the exercises.

How to Avoid It:

- **Breathe Normally**: Ensure you breathe deeply and normally throughout each exercise.

- **Coordinate Breathing**: Inhale when relaxing the pelvic floor muscles and exhale when contracting them. This helps maintain a steady breathing pattern.

Mistake 3: Overdoing It

Description: Overworking the pelvic floor muscles by doing too many repetitions or holding contractions for too long can lead to muscle fatigue and potential injury.

How to Avoid It:

- **Follow a Routine**: Stick to the recommended number of repetitions and sets outlined in previous chapters.

- **Listen to Your Body**: Pay attention to how your muscles feel. If you experience fatigue or discomfort, reduce the number of repetitions or take a break.

Mistake 4: Inconsistent Practice

Description: Inconsistency in performing pelvic floor exercises can lead to minimal or no improvements.

How to Avoid It:

- **Set a Schedule**: Incorporate pelvic floor exercises into your daily routine as outlined in Chapter 6.

- **Use Reminders**: Set reminders on your phone or place visual cues around your home to prompt you to do your exercises.

- **Track Your Progress**: Keep a journal or use an app to

monitor your consistency and progress.

Mistake 5: Lack of Progression

Description: Sticking to the same basic exercises without progressing to more advanced movements can limit improvements.

How to Avoid It:

- **Advance Gradually**: Once you have mastered basic exercises, move on to more advanced exercises as discussed in Chapter 5.

- **Increase Repetitions and Duration**: Gradually increase the number of repetitions and the duration of holds as your strength improves.

- **Challenge Yourself**: Introduce new variations and challenges to keep your routine effective and engaging.

Mistake 6: Ignoring Other Muscle Groups

Description: Focusing solely on the pelvic floor muscles without incorporating other core and lower body exercises can lead to an imbalance.

How to Avoid It:

- **Integrate Full-Body Exercises**: Include exercises that engage multiple muscle groups, such as squats and bridge poses, into your routine.

- **Balance Your Workouts**: Ensure your fitness regimen includes a variety of exercises that strengthen the core, glutes, and legs.

Mistake 7: Not Seeking Professional Guidance

Description: Attempting to perform pelvic floor exercises without proper guidance can lead to incorrect techniques and reduced effectiveness.

How to Avoid It:

- **Consult a Professional**: If you're unsure about your technique or experiencing difficulties, seek advice from a physical therapist or fitness instructor with experience in pelvic health.

- **Attend Workshops or Classes**: Participate in pelvic floor exercise classes or workshops to learn proper techniques and receive personalized feedback.

Common Mistake Correction Summary

- **Isolate the Correct Muscles**: Focus solely on the pelvic floor muscles.

- **Breathe Properly**: Maintain normal, coordinated breathing throughout exercises.

- **Avoid Overworking**: Stick to recommended repetitions and listen to your body.

- **Be Consistent**: Make pelvic floor exercises a regular part of your daily routine.

- **Progress Gradually**: Move from basic to advanced exercises as your strength improves.

- **Engage Multiple Muscles**: Incorporate full-body exercises to maintain balance.

- **Seek Professional Help**: Consult with experts for proper guidance and technique.

By being aware of these common mistakes and taking steps to avoid them, you can maximize the effectiveness of your pelvic floor exercises. Consistent, correct practice will lead to stronger pelvic floor muscles, improved bladder and bowel control, enhanced sexual function, and overall better pelvic health.

CHAPTER 8:
ADDITIONAL TIPS
FOR PELVIC HEALTH

In addition to regular exercises, maintaining optimal pelvic health involves several lifestyle changes, dietary adjustments, and habits. This chapter provides comprehensive tips to support your pelvic health beyond exercises, ensuring a holistic approach to well-being.

Lifestyle Changes

1. **Maintain a Healthy Weight**: Excess weight puts additional pressure on the pelvic floor muscles. Maintaining a healthy weight through a balanced diet and regular physical activity can help reduce this strain.

2. **Stay Active**: Engage in regular physical activity such as walking, swimming, or cycling. Staying active helps keep your muscles, including the pelvic floor muscles, strong and functional.

3. **Avoid Heavy Lifting**: When lifting heavy objects, use proper techniques to avoid straining your pelvic floor muscles. Bend at the knees and keep the object close to your body. Exhale while lifting to reduce intra-abdominal pressure.

4. **Practice Good Posture**: Maintaining good posture helps support your pelvic floor. Sit and stand with a straight

back, shoulders back, and pelvis in a neutral position.

5. **Quit Smoking**: Smoking can lead to chronic coughing, which puts pressure on the pelvic floor muscles. Quitting smoking can improve overall health and reduce pelvic floor strain.

Dietary Adjustments

1. **Stay Hydrated**: Drink plenty of water throughout the day to stay hydrated and maintain healthy bladder function. Aim for 6-8 glasses of water daily.

2. **Eat a High-Fiber Diet**: Consuming a diet rich in fiber helps prevent constipation, which can strain the pelvic floor muscles. Include plenty of fruits, vegetables, whole grains, and legumes in your diet.

3. **Limit Caffeine and Alcohol**: Both caffeine and alcohol can irritate the bladder and lead to increased urgency and frequency of urination. Limiting their intake can help improve bladder control.

4. **Manage Bladder Irritants**: Some foods and beverages, such as spicy foods, citrus fruits, and carbonated drinks, can irritate the bladder. Monitor your diet to identify and reduce intake of these irritants.

Healthy Habits

1. **Practice Bladder Training**: Gradually increase the time between bathroom visits to train your bladder to hold more urine. This can help reduce urgency and frequency issues.

2. **Empty Your Bladder Completely**: Take your time to fully empty your bladder when urinating. This can help prevent urinary tract infections and ensure that no urine is left behind.

3. **Avoid Straining During Bowel Movements**: Use proper techniques to avoid straining during bowel movements.

Relax and give yourself time. If necessary, use a stool to elevate your feet and promote easier bowel movements.

4. **Use Proper Lifting Techniques**: When lifting objects, bend your knees, keep your back straight, and avoid holding your breath. Exhale as you lift to reduce pressure on your pelvic floor.

5. **Manage Stress**: High stress levels can affect your overall health, including your pelvic floor muscles. Practice stress-relieving techniques such as deep breathing, meditation, or yoga.

6. **Wear Supportive Clothing**: Avoid tight clothing that can put pressure on your pelvic area. Opt for comfortable, supportive clothing that allows for better movement and reduces strain on your pelvic floor.

Regular Check-Ups

1. **Visit Your Healthcare Provider**: Regular check-ups with your healthcare provider can help monitor your pelvic health and address any issues early on. Discuss any symptoms or concerns you may have.

2. **Seek Professional Advice**: If you experience persistent pelvic floor issues, consider consulting a pelvic health specialist or physical therapist. They can provide personalized advice and treatment options.

3. **Stay Informed**: Keep yourself informed about pelvic health by reading reliable sources and staying updated on new research and techniques. Knowledge is key to maintaining good health.

Integrating Tips into Your Routine

To make these tips a part of your daily life, consider the following strategies:

- **Create a Plan**: Develop a comprehensive plan that includes your exercise routine, dietary adjustments, and lifestyle changes. Write down your goals and steps to achieve them.

- **Use Technology**: Utilize apps and digital reminders to keep track of your hydration, diet, and exercise routine. Technology can help you stay organized and consistent.

- **Build a Support System**: Share your goals with family and friends. Having a support system can provide encouragement and accountability.

- **Make Gradual Changes**: Implement changes gradually to avoid feeling overwhelmed. Small, consistent steps can lead to significant improvements over time.

By incorporating these additional tips into your daily life, you can enhance the benefits of your pelvic floor exercises and maintain overall pelvic health. A holistic approach that includes lifestyle changes, dietary adjustments, and healthy habits will help you achieve long-term well-being and improve your quality of life.

CHAPTER 9: CONCLUSION AND MOVING FORWARD

As we reach the conclusion of this guide, it's essential to reflect on the journey we've undertaken to understand and improve pelvic floor health. This final chapter will summarize the key points and offer encouragement to continue practicing pelvic floor exercises regularly, emphasizing their long-term benefits.

Summary of Key Points

1. **Importance of Pelvic Floor Muscles**:
   - Pelvic floor muscles are crucial for maintaining the health and function of the bladder, bowels, and sexual organs.
   - Keeping these muscles strong and healthy can prevent various issues, such as incontinence and pelvic organ prolapse.

2. **Benefits of Pelvic Floor Exercises**:
   - Improved bladder and bowel control.
   - Enhanced sexual function and satisfaction.
   - Reduced risk of pelvic organ prolapse.
   - Overall improved core stability and strength.

3. **Understanding the Pelvic Floor**:
   - The pelvic floor consists of layers of muscles and tissues that provide support to pelvic

organs.

- Knowing the anatomy and function of these muscles is essential for effective exercise.

4. **Basic Pelvic Floor Exercises**:
   - Kegel Exercises: The foundation of pelvic floor workouts, focusing on contraction and relaxation.
   - Quick Flick Kegels: Quick, short contractions to build strength and endurance.
   - Long Hold Kegels: Extended contractions to enhance muscle control.

5. **Advanced Pelvic Floor Exercises**:
   - Bridge Pose: Targets the pelvic floor, glutes, and lower back.
   - Squats: Engage the pelvic floor, thighs, and glutes.
   - Split Tabletop: An advanced exercise requiring balance and engaging multiple muscle groups.

6. **Integrating Exercises into Daily Life**:
   - Making pelvic floor exercises a habit through reminders and associating them with daily activities.
   - Incorporating exercises into your routine and staying consistent.

7. **Common Mistakes and How to Avoid Them**:
   - Incorrect muscle engagement, holding breath, overdoing it, and inconsistent practice.
   - Progressing gradually, engaging multiple muscles, and seeking professional guidance.

8. **Additional Tips for Pelvic Health**:
   - Lifestyle changes, dietary adjustments, and healthy habits.

- Maintaining a healthy weight, staying active, avoiding heavy lifting, and practicing good posture.
- Regular check-ups and professional advice for personalized care.

Encouragement to Continue

Maintaining a consistent routine of pelvic floor exercises is vital for long-term benefits. Here are some motivational tips to help you stay committed:

1. **Celebrate Small Wins**: Recognize and celebrate your progress, no matter how small. Each improvement is a step towards better pelvic health.

2. **Set Realistic Goals**: Establish achievable goals and work towards them gradually. Clear objectives can keep you motivated and focused.

3. **Stay Positive**: Keep a positive mindset and be patient with yourself. Progress might be slow, but perseverance will lead to success.

4. **Incorporate Variety**: Keep your routine interesting by incorporating different exercises and variations. This prevents monotony and keeps you engaged.

5. **Seek Support**: Share your journey with friends, family, or a support group. Having a network of encouragement can boost your motivation.

Moving Forward

As you move forward, remember that pelvic floor health is an ongoing journey. The benefits of strong pelvic floor muscles extend beyond physical health, contributing to overall well-being and quality of life. By consistently practicing the exercises and integrating the additional tips into your lifestyle, you can achieve and maintain optimal pelvic health.

Continue to educate yourself, seek professional guidance when needed, and stay committed to your routine. Your efforts will pay off, leading to improved control, strength, and confidence.

Thank you for taking the time to read this guide and for your dedication to improving your pelvic health. Here's to a healthier, stronger, and more confident you!